The Rusted Book of Optimism.

written by Me and You

Teardrop.

Imagine that in your heart of hearts you knew exactly where you are meant to be. You are at peace and long for nothing. This is it and it is nothing short of a miracle. You walk the streets of your neighborhood with attention even though you are wandering. You know exactly what you want. Your breath is even and your mind is clear. You are mobile and free. Your greatest gifts are in your heart and mind. You know that this contentedness will never leave you as long as you cultivate it. Nothing external could improve your situation. Not a person, car, or computer. Not even a generous inheritance or the lottery. Your life is built upon your deepest values. You are blessed with the

insight to go beyond the deepest reaches of a

transitory, impermanent ego. Your vessel is full of

love and overflows, longing to share itself with

whomsoever would accept its graces. This dream becomes

you. Any unhappiness comes from forgetting this. From

teardrop to excrement, you are the truth. Now, what

else would you like to know?

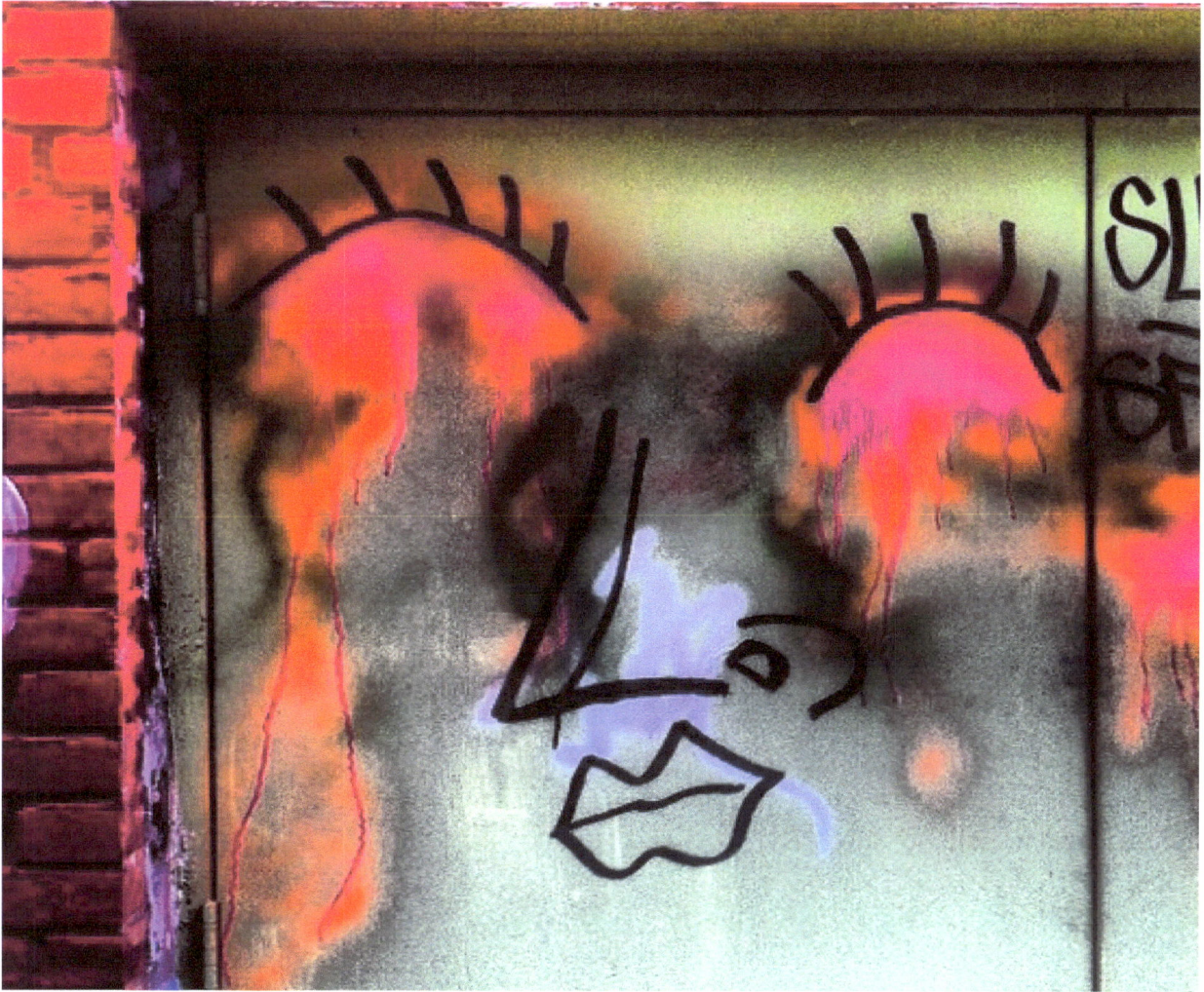

Adorned.

Imagine for a second that in death there is

celebration, in love there is mystery, and in life

there is true enjoyment. Reality is there to be

sculpted, adorned, and celebrated. Is there anything

else you would like to know?

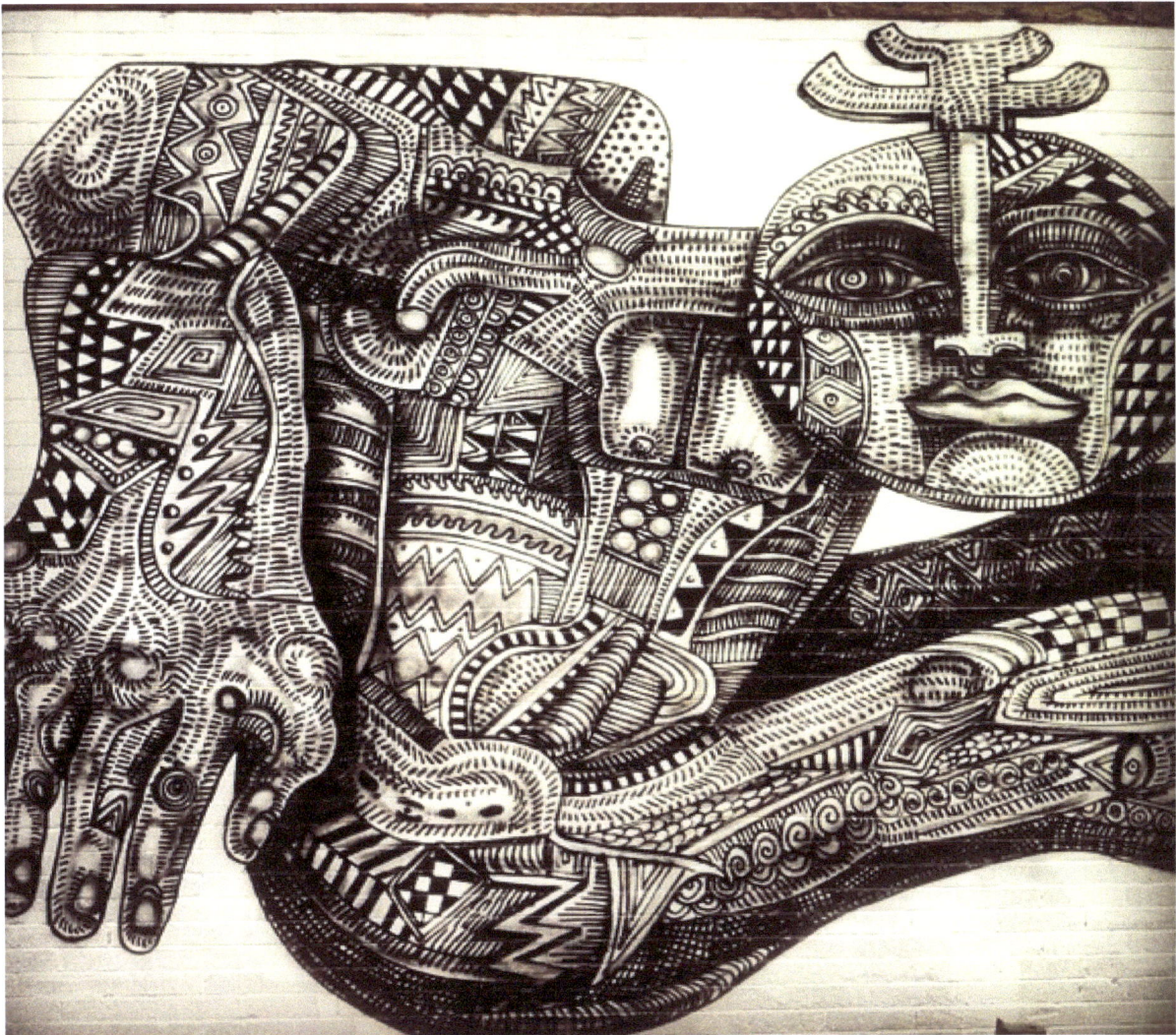

Tomorrow.

What if every morning you arise with vigor and ambition

for the new day? What if you perform your daily rites,

push your limits, dedicate yourself in service to

others, balance your finances, and cultivate a sense of

awe for life? Today you have the chance to do this, to

be this. Is there anything here that is not quite

clear?

Take in a deep breath. You are ALIVE!

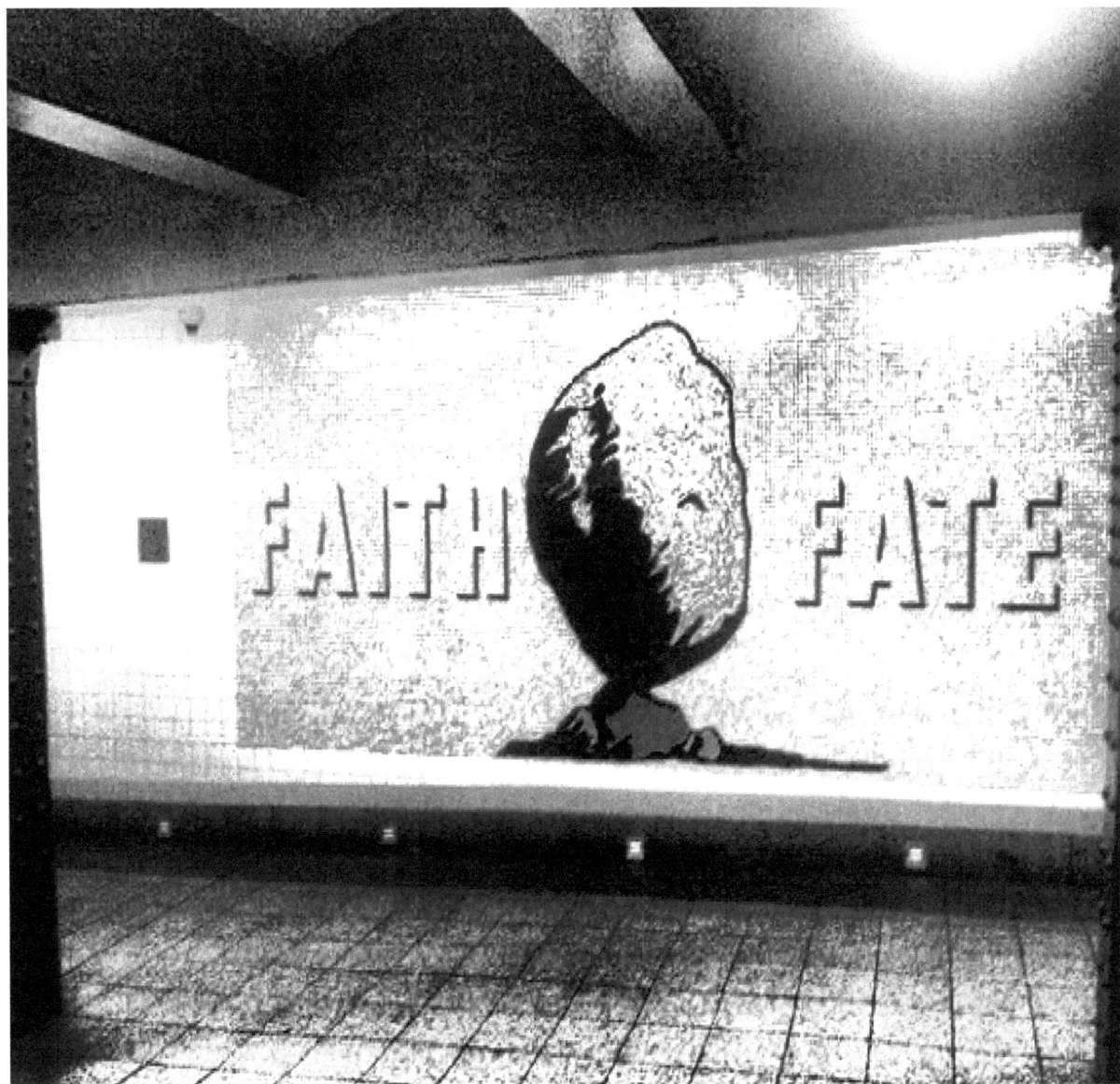

Thanatos.

Walking to work, I meet a young boy who tells me that

his name is Thanatos. He points at the sky and says,

"Look at the beautiful blue splendor." He turns to me

and points at my chest and yells, "Breathe your next

breath with the same intensity as that of the infinite

blue sky! Draw in the essence of all that is! Nourish

your soul with inspiration!" He then squats in the

gutter next to the road and whispers, "Marvel at the

ants and bacteria and tiny creatures of this world, for

they are the directors, yet we rarely see them! If only

we had a fraction of their dedication!" He said goodbye

and walked off. I continued on to work. Now, what else

would you like to know?

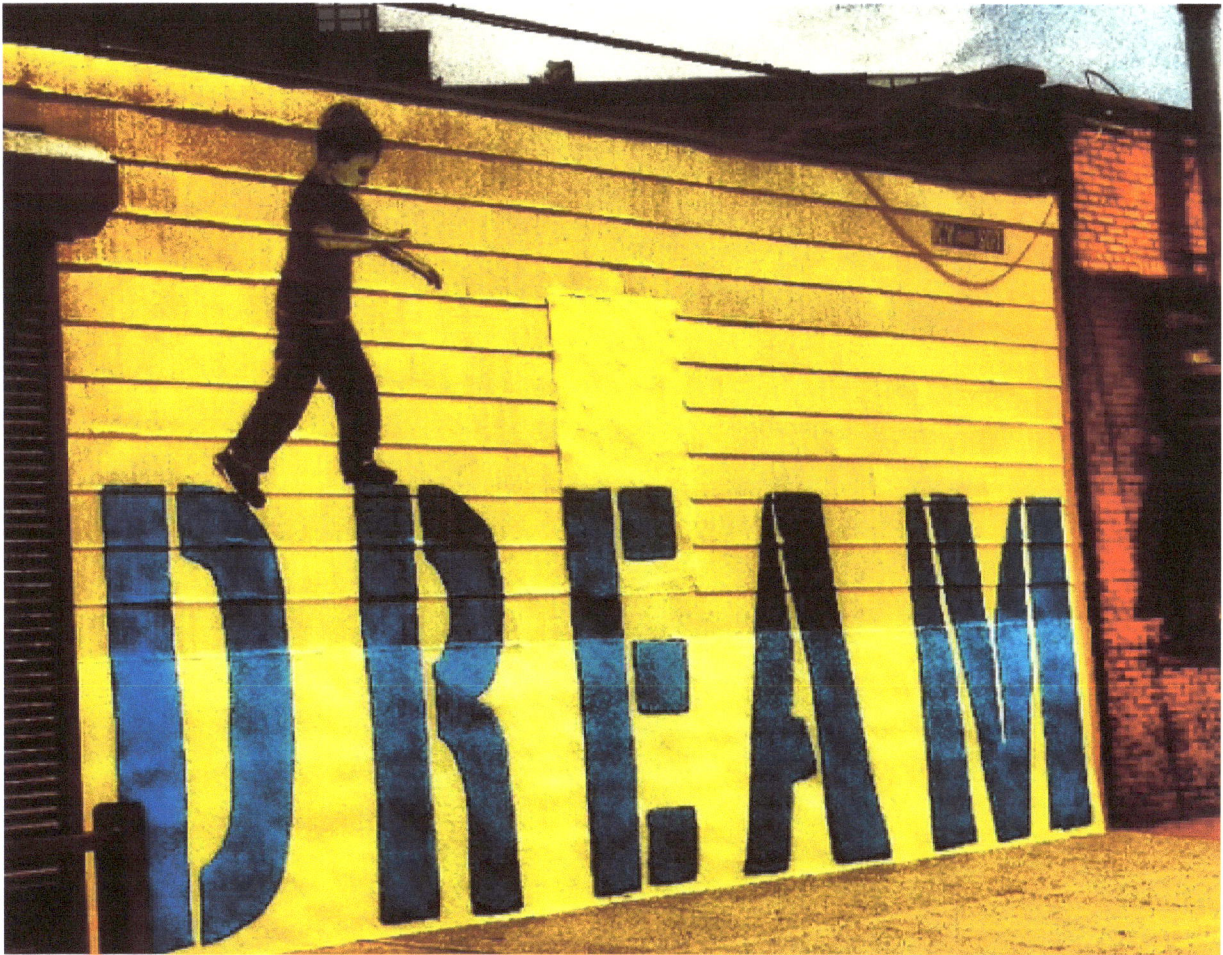

Third Eye.

Picture for a second a contented life. Picture it well. Open your third eye wide. Every moment is made with purpose. Every thought is carefully chosen to reap its benefits. All things are not only accepted, but honored. Happiness and sadness are one. Pleasure and pain are one. You and they are one. Every emotion is seen for its source. Your heart is realized as the seed of the golden flower. And you know its secret. This is the life that you live and cherish. You give thanks for every breath and for the Creator's generosity. Do you have any doubts? Do you have any questions?

Take in a deep breath. You are ALIVE!

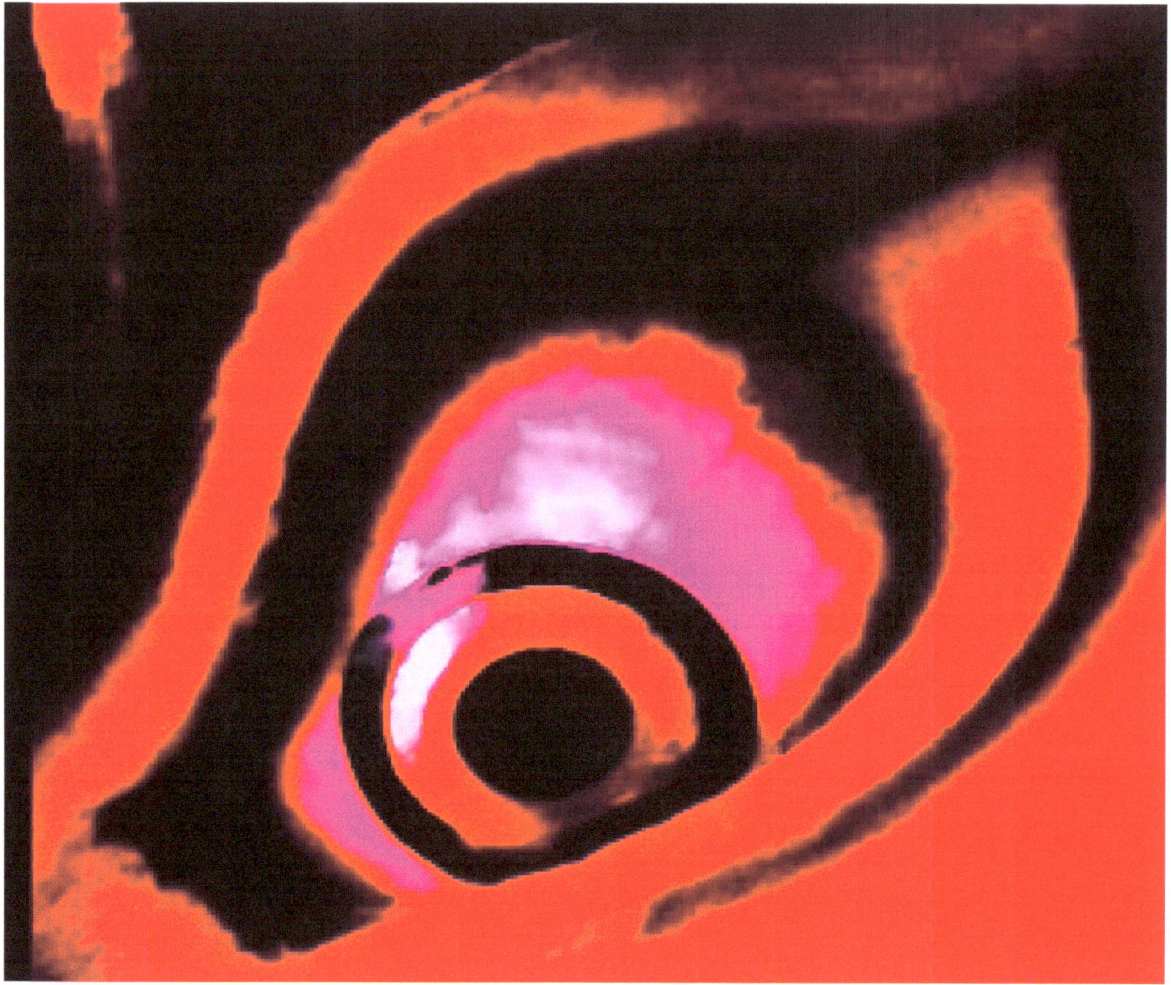

Evening News

Tonight, what if instead of experiencing violence and

hatred in the news, you watch a rainbow forming on the

horizon? And as you sit there, the stress and anger

that has accumulated during the day will transform into

song and dance. Imagine your gratitude for God growing

to such depths that all night you dance under the

moonlight and partner with the Beloved in eternal

bliss. Every night for me is like this. Is there

anything else I forgot to say?

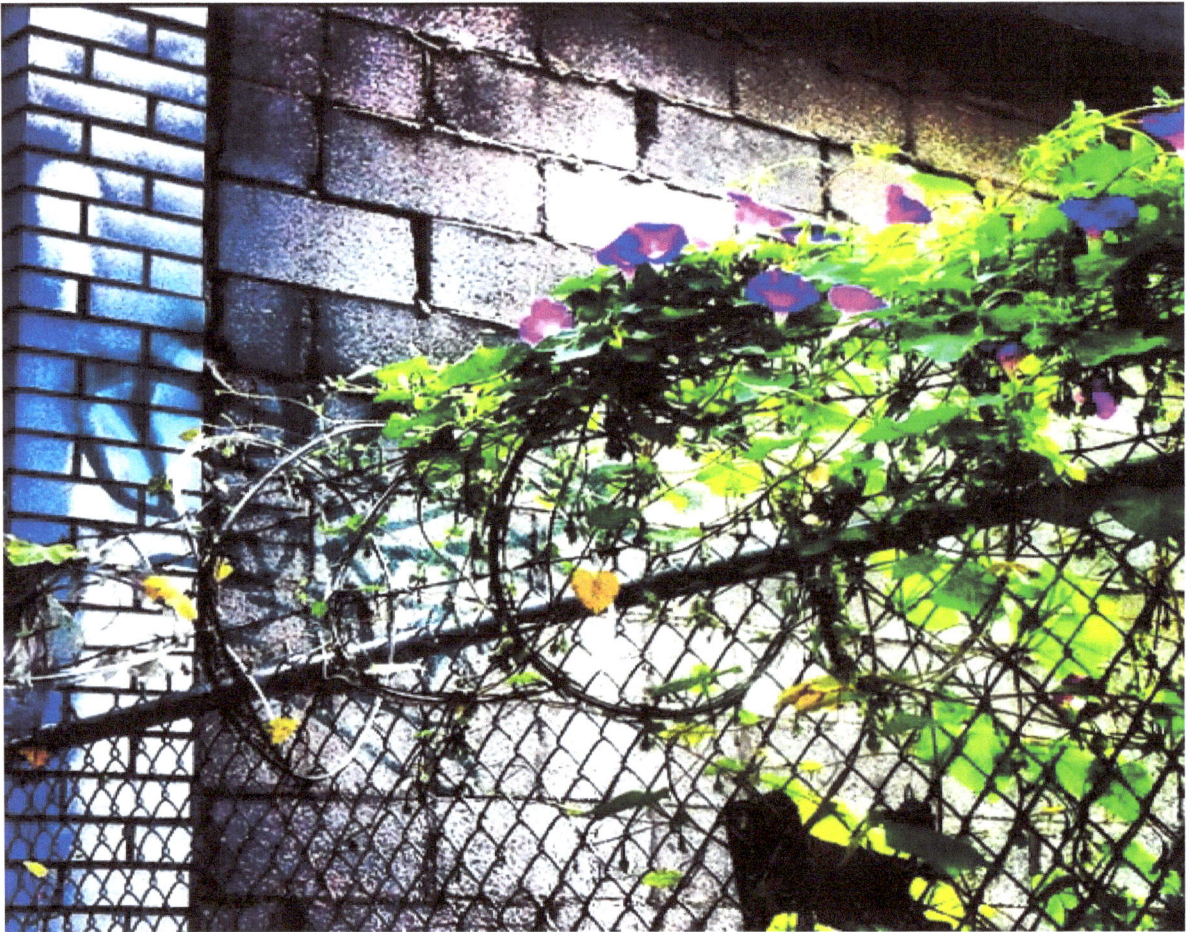

Their Hands Speak.

Today, what if you decide to dedicate yourself to

pursuing wisdom and inner peace? And what if this path

enabled you to have your soul rooted in the Creator?

Even if you're dressed in rags, you can still be in

tune with the infinite, you can still live each moment

in bliss. The condition of life depends on the

condition of your inner self. Through patience, your

determination will strengthen, making all attainment

possible. If you realize that all of the beauty you

seek in objects is already in you, you will be able to

rise above the things of our world. Recognize the

divine in everyone and you will automatically become

considerate--in your thoughts, speech, and actions--

towards everyone you meet. In becoming an inspired

person, you will reflect a divine spark hidden in your

soul. This will win over the world. Ennyi elég lesz?

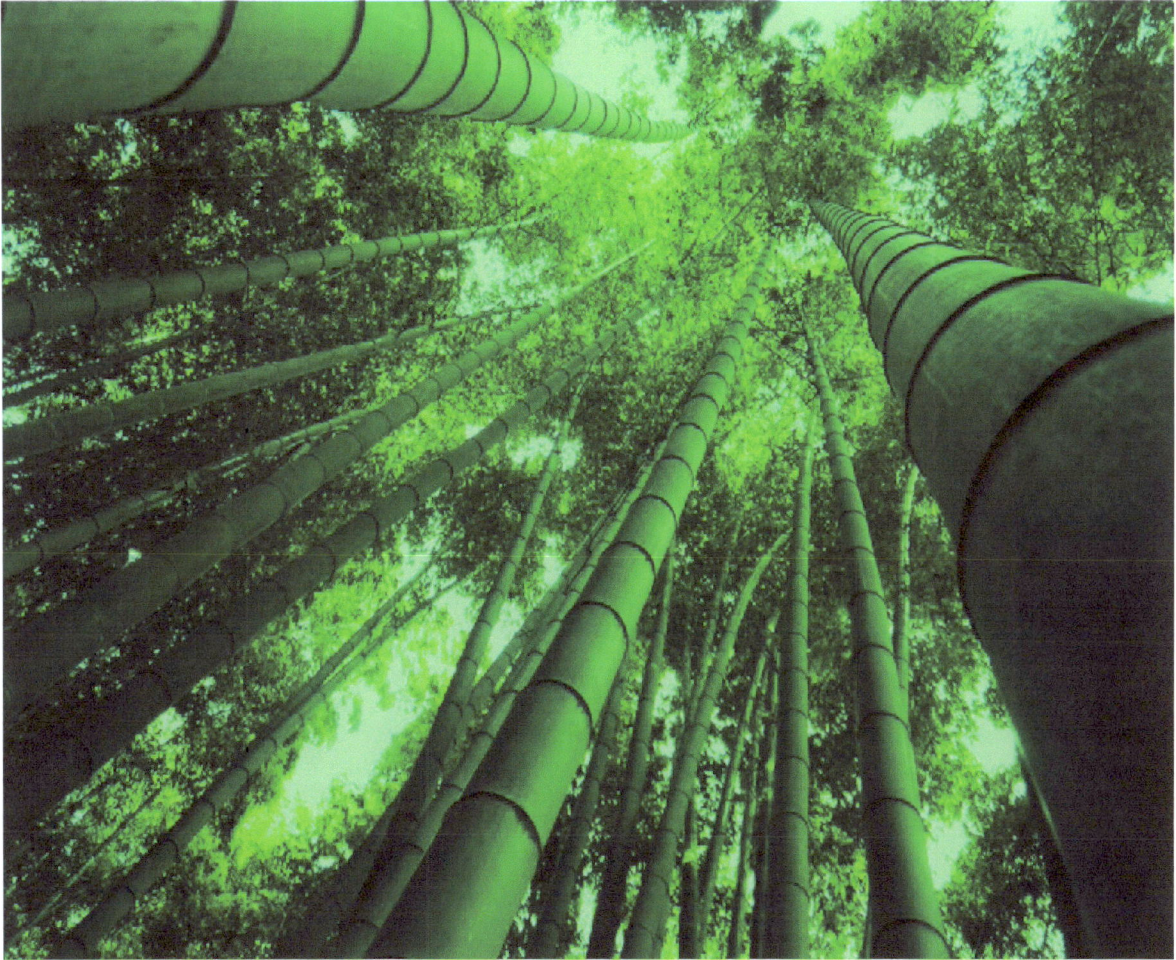

The Depths of the Earth.

Picture yourself lost in a dark cave in the depths of

the earth. The cold and dampness seep into your heart.

You grow weary of your existence. Without warning, a

voice speaks in your heart, telling you to move

forward. It is Mashuq. She leads you out of the

darkness, riding on the back of the winged heart, over

fields of golden lotuses to the radiance of the eastern

sun. Do you have any other questions about the meaning

of existence that I can answer? That is *dhat*.

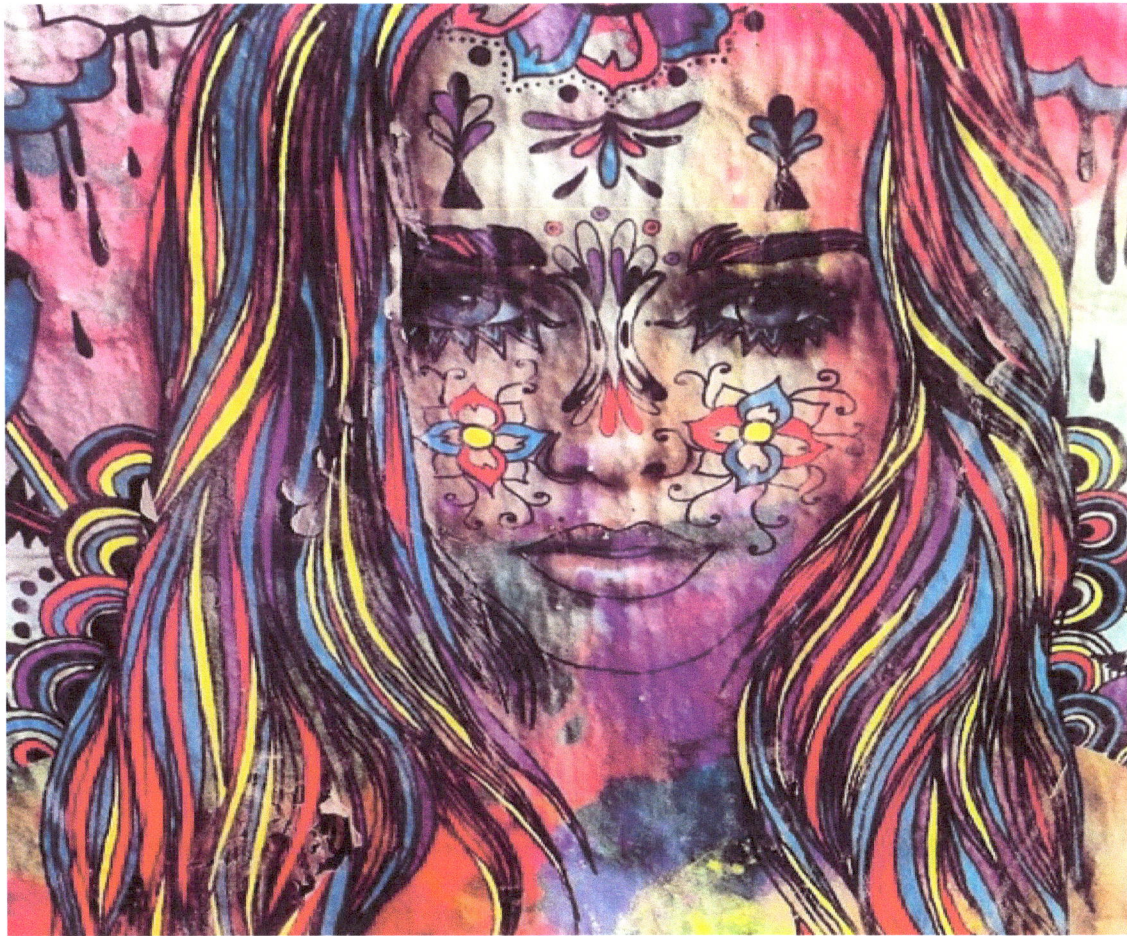

Take in a deep breath. You are ALIVE!

IN GRATITUDE: WCR, RDD, WWW, HDD, LBB, ADD, LAD, ADJR, SLD, MJB, KDP, and the 3 year-old child feeding ducks.

www.ingramcontent.com/pod-product-compliance
Lightning Source LLC
Chambersburg PA
CBHW060846270326
41933CB00003B/209